For My Boys

J.R., who's watching over us

&

Theo, who's growing stronger every day

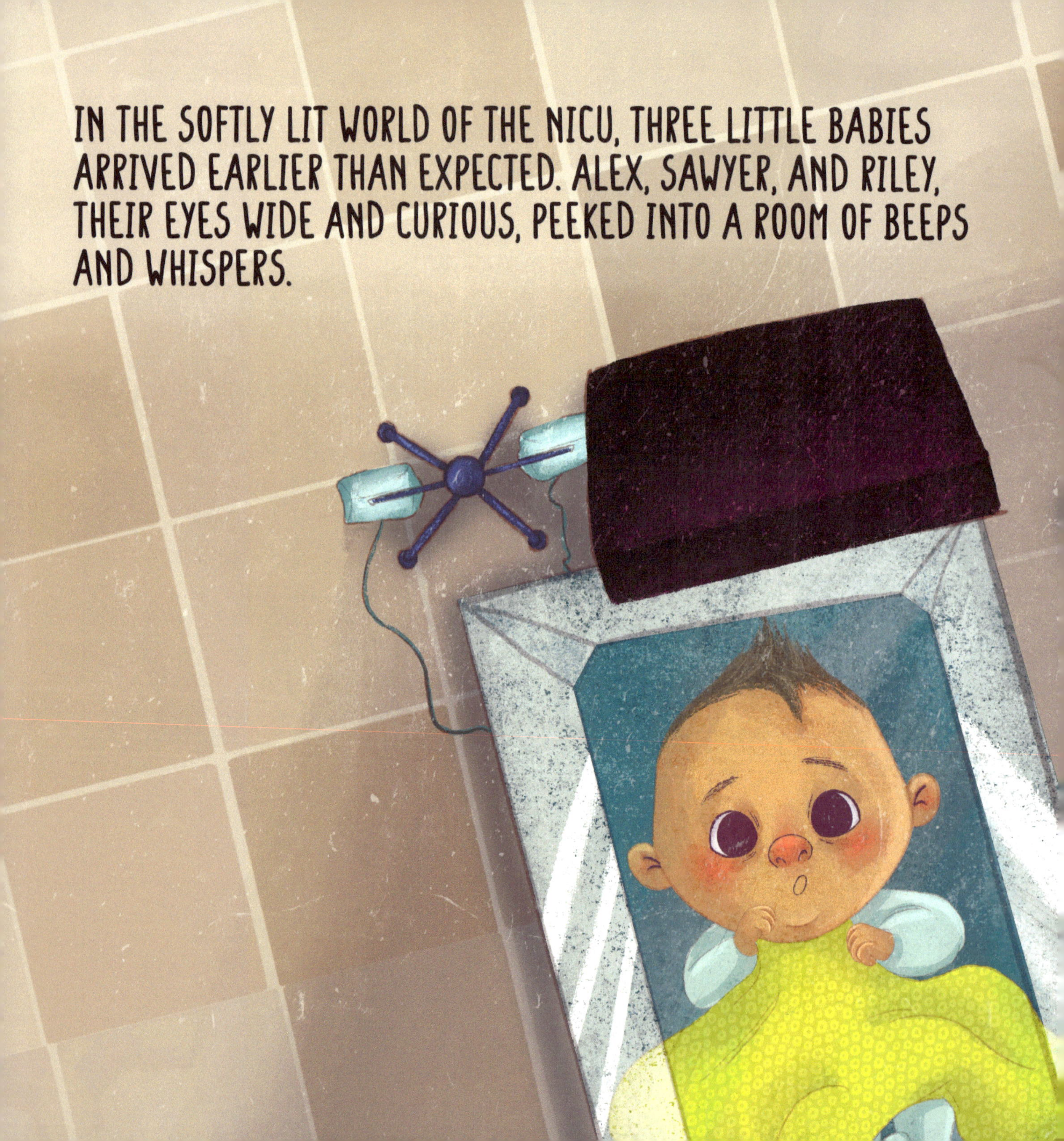

IN THE SOFTLY LIT WORLD OF THE NICU, THREE LITTLE BABIES ARRIVED EARLIER THAN EXPECTED. ALEX, SAWYER, AND RILEY, THEIR EYES WIDE AND CURIOUS, PEEKED INTO A ROOM OF BEEPS AND WHISPERS.

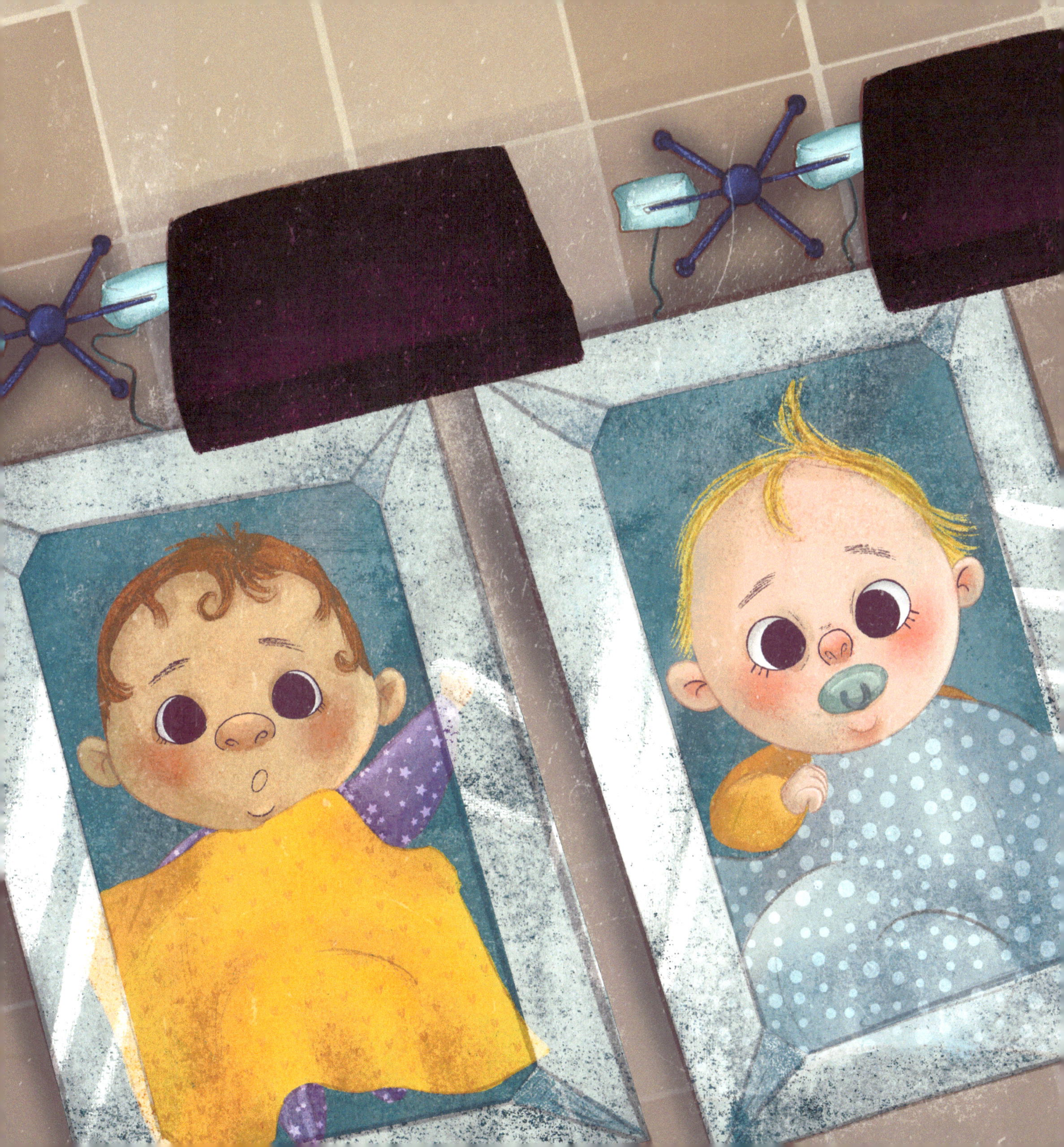

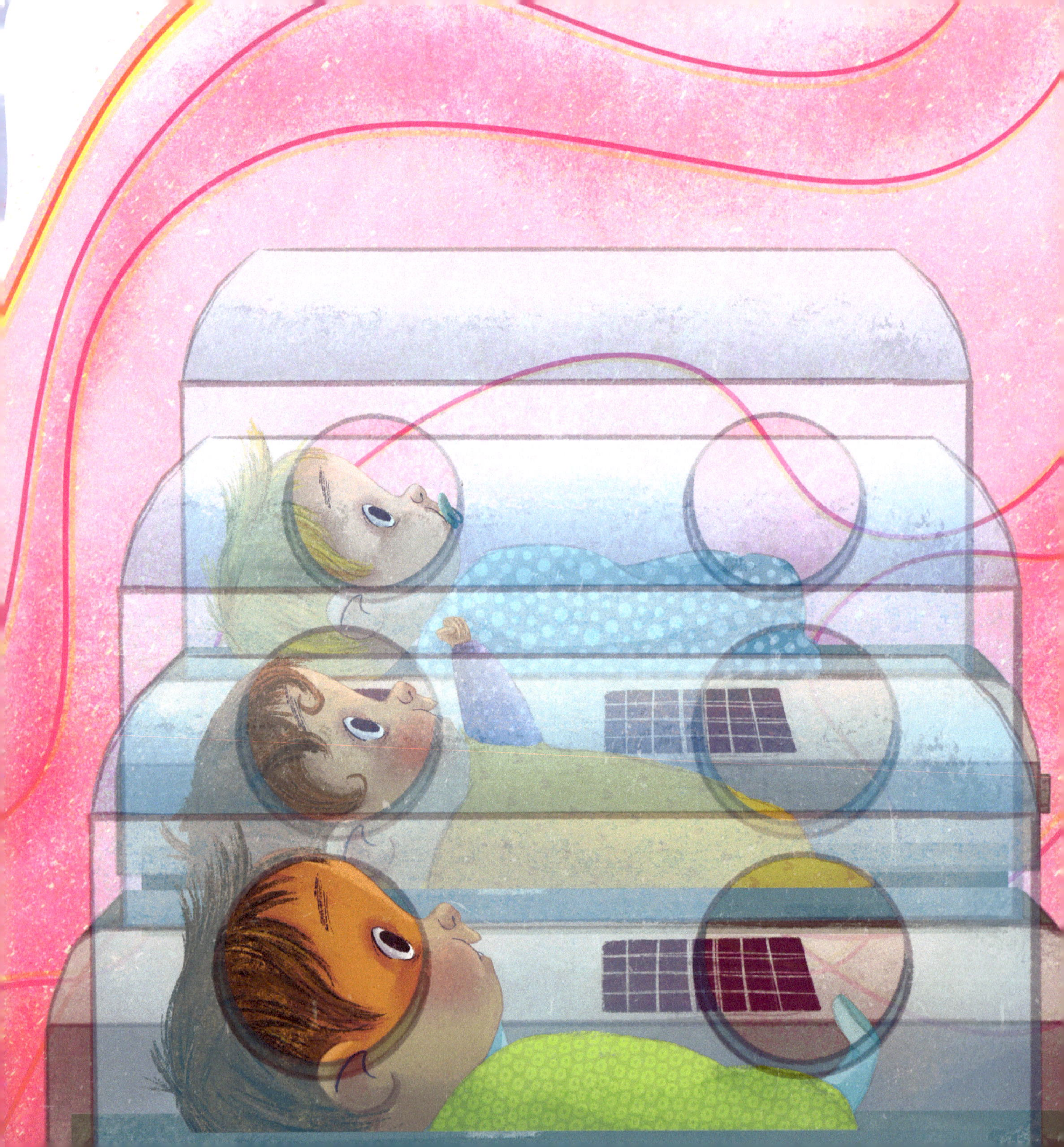

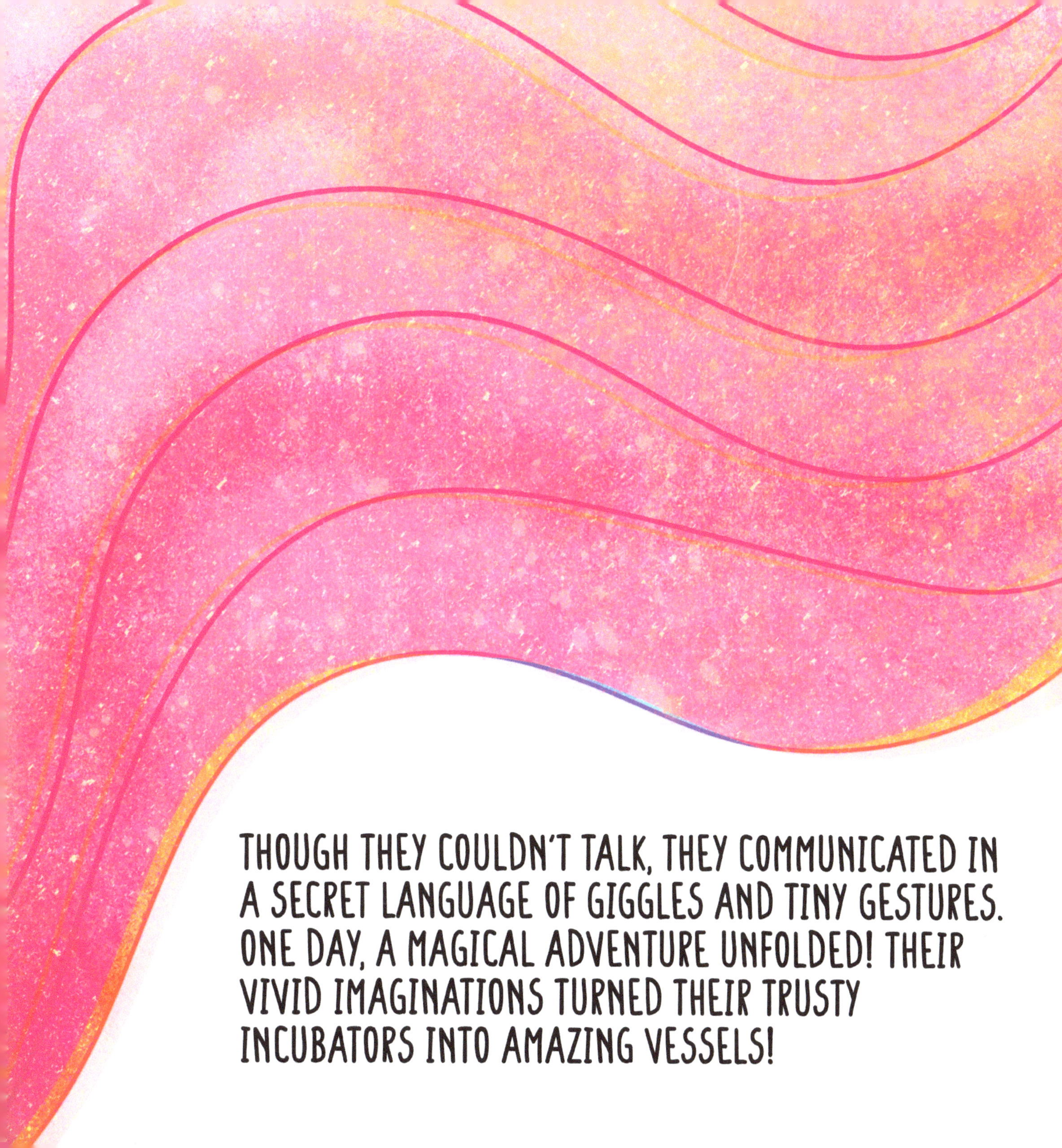

THOUGH THEY COULDN'T TALK, THEY COMMUNICATED IN
A SECRET LANGUAGE OF GIGGLES AND TINY GESTURES.
ONE DAY, A MAGICAL ADVENTURE UNFOLDED! THEIR
VIVID IMAGINATIONS TURNED THEIR TRUSTY
INCUBATORS INTO AMAZING VESSELS!

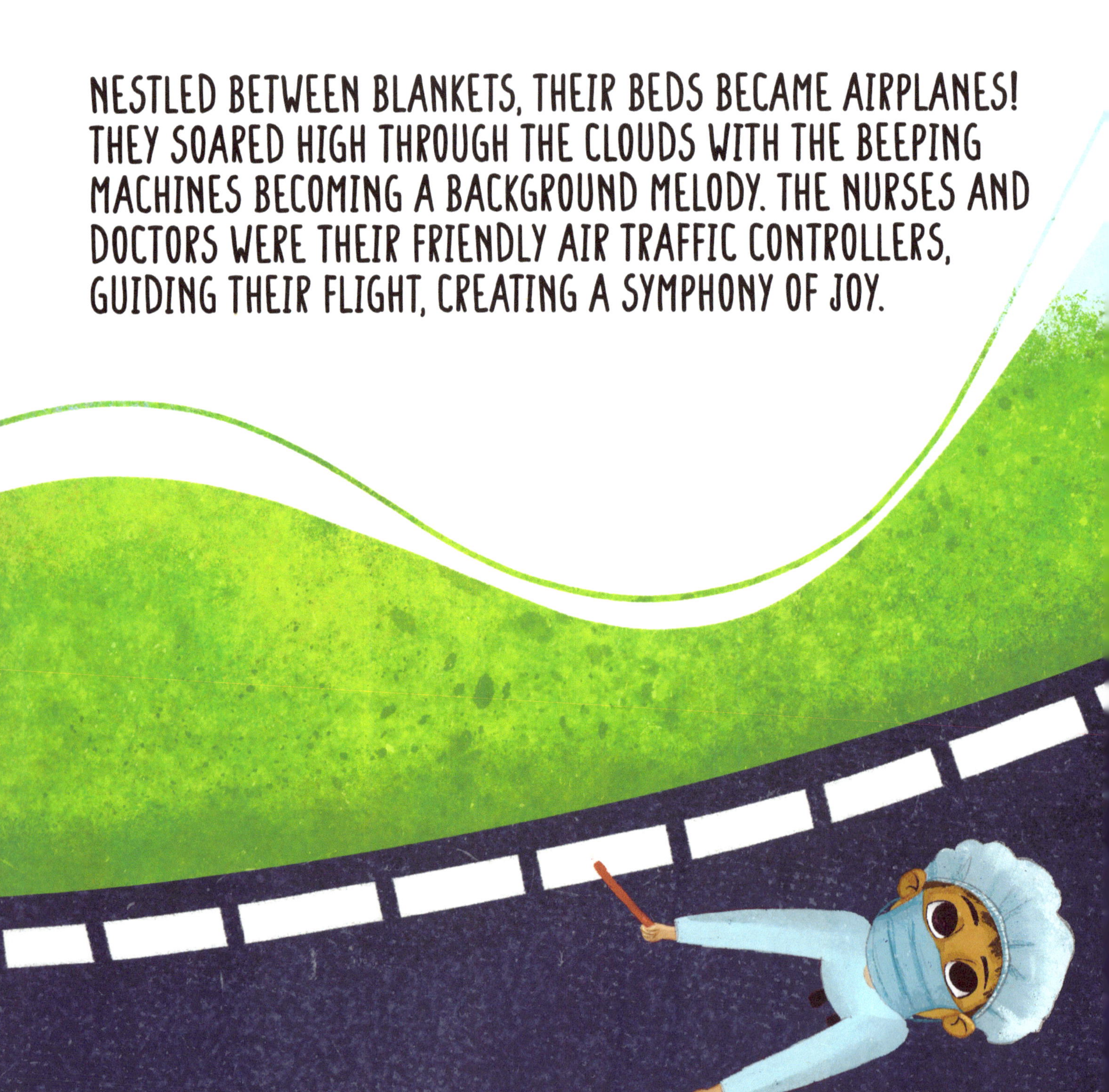

NESTLED BETWEEN BLANKETS, THEIR BEDS BECAME AIRPLANES! THEY SOARED HIGH THROUGH THE CLOUDS WITH THE BEEPING MACHINES BECOMING A BACKGROUND MELODY. THE NURSES AND DOCTORS WERE THEIR FRIENDLY AIR TRAFFIC CONTROLLERS, GUIDING THEIR FLIGHT, CREATING A SYMPHONY OF JOY.

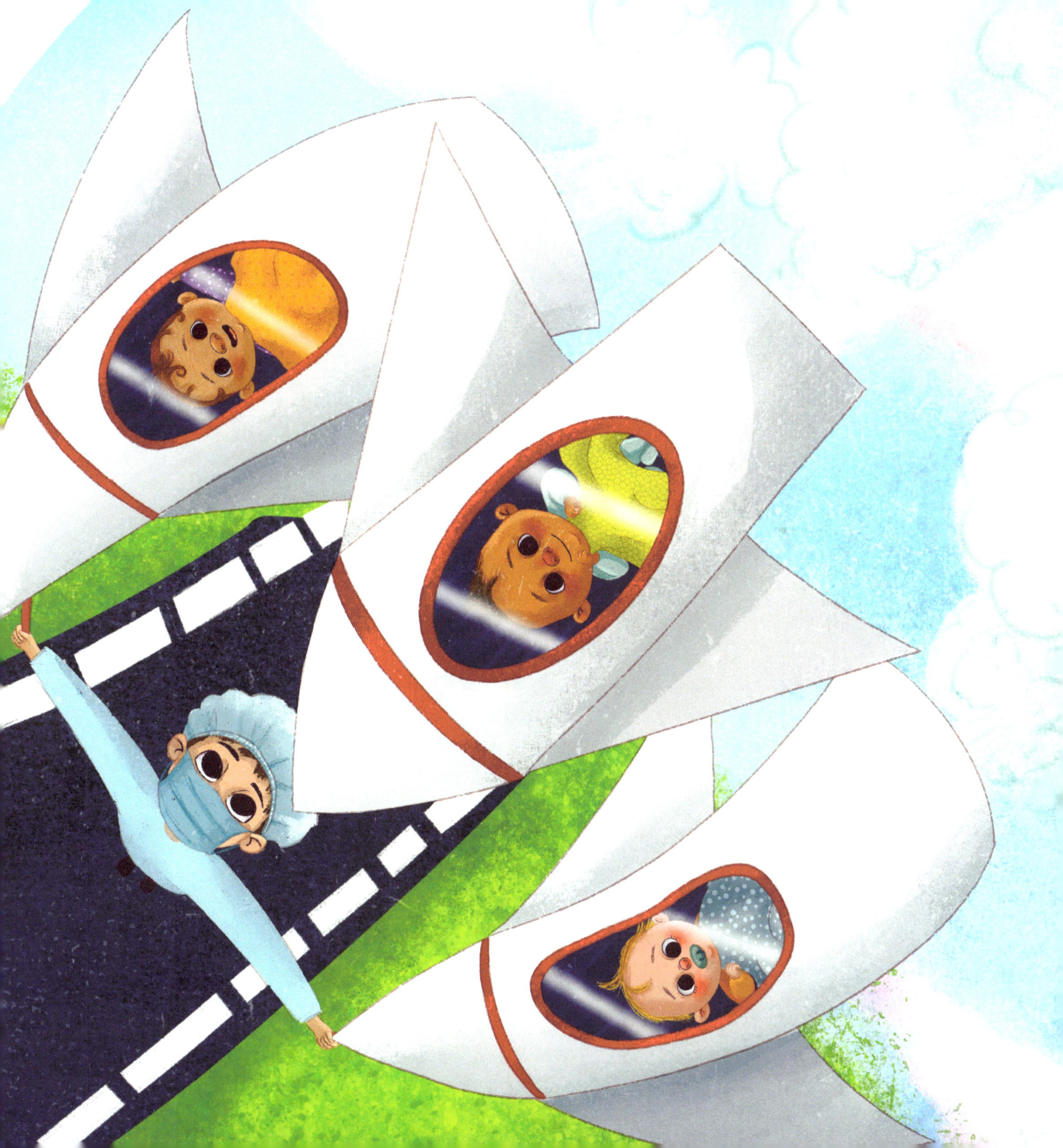

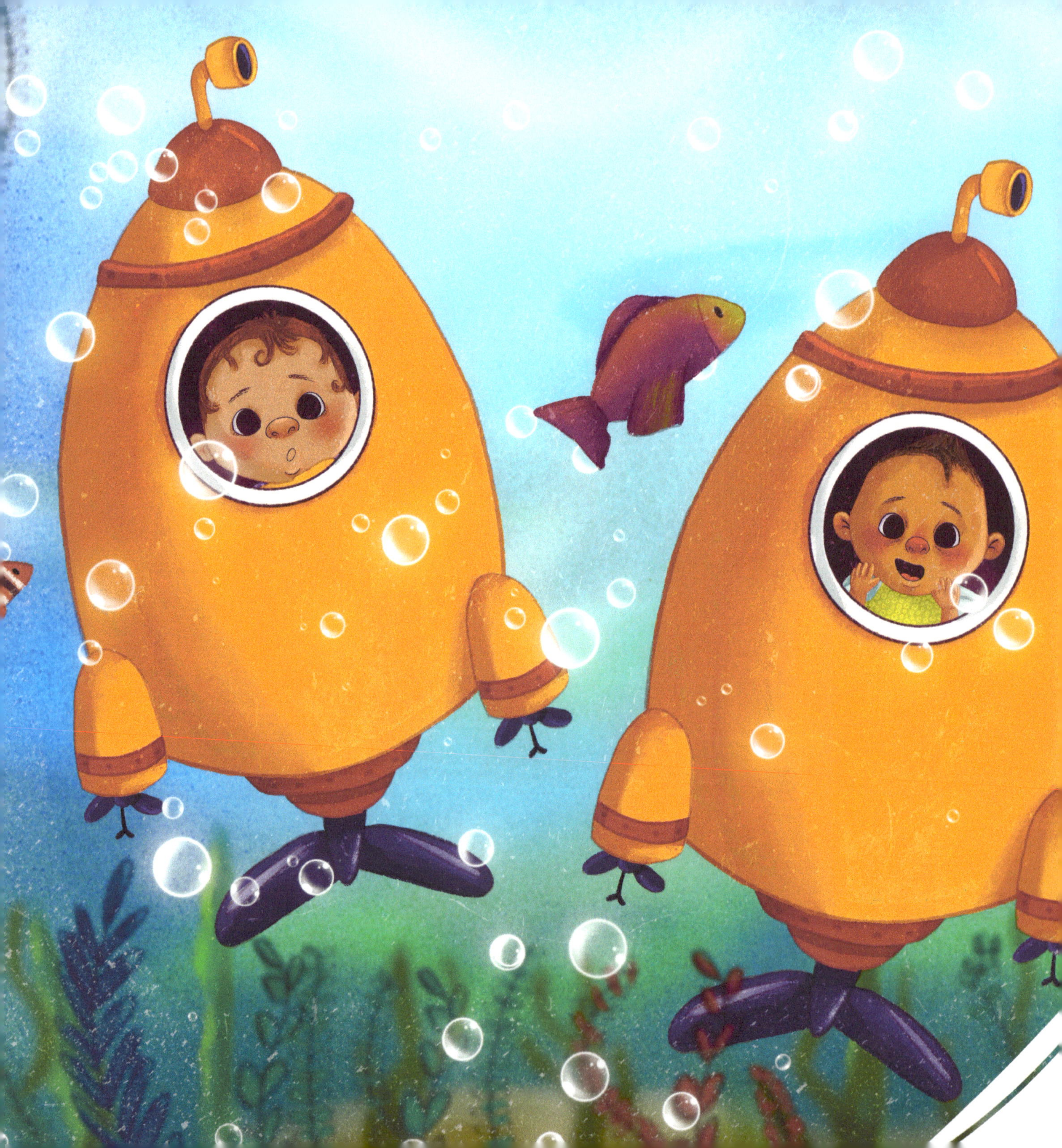

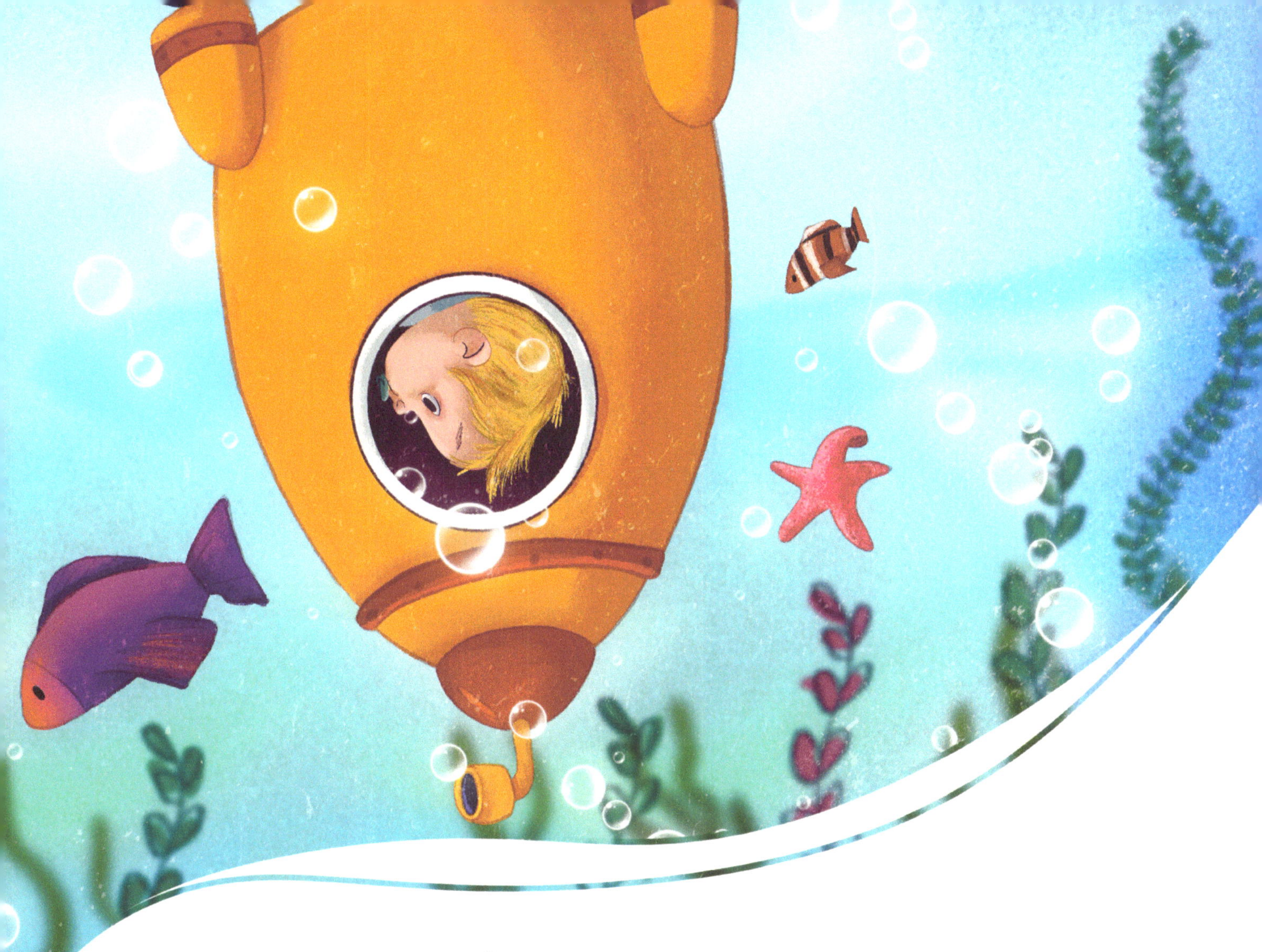

NEXT, THE THREE ADVENTURERS DESCENDED INTO THE DEPTHS INSIDE TINY SUBMARINES! THE BEEPING SOUNDS TRANSFORMING TO SONAR ECHOES OF UNDERWATER EXPLORATION. THE ROOM, ONCE QUIET WITH HUSHED TONES, NOW ECHOED WITH THE LAUGHTER OF BABIES ON A MAGICAL VOYAGE, FINDING HIDDEN TREASURE IN THE DEEP BLUE SEA.

THEIR ADVENTURE CONTINUED, AND THE TINY CREW BOARDED THEIR
TINY SPACESHIPS! THE BEEPING MONITORS BLENDED IN WITH THE
HUM OF THE POWERFUL ENGINES. THE NURSES AND DOCTORS SAT IN
MISSION CONTROL AND SAID "GO FOR LAUNCH!"
IN THIS COSMIC ADVENTURE, THE SMALL ROOM BECAME A
PORTAL TO DISTANT GALAXIES, AND THE THREE FRIENDS
FLOATED WEIGHTLESSLY AMONG THE STARS
WITHIN THEIR COZY BEDS.

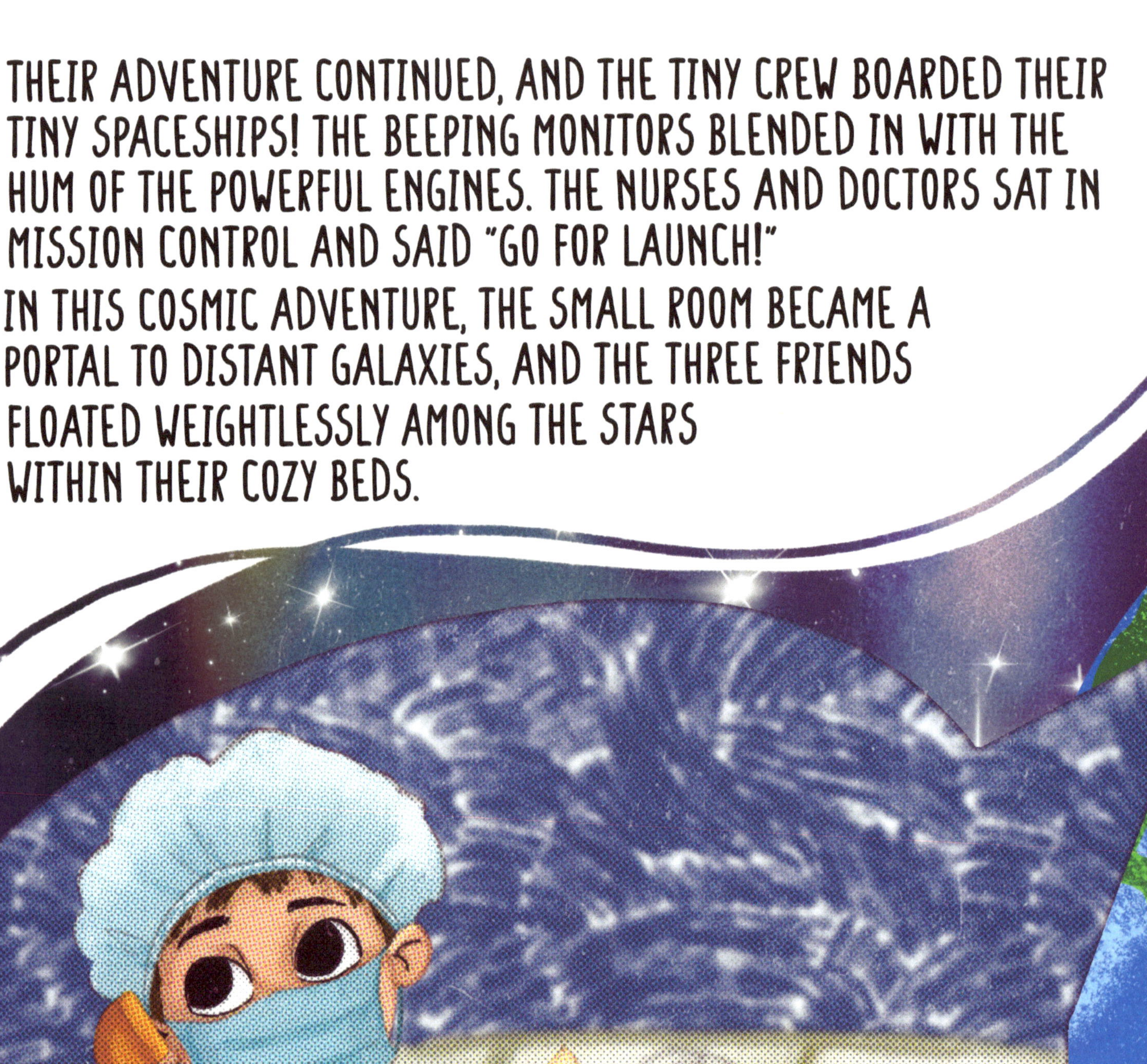

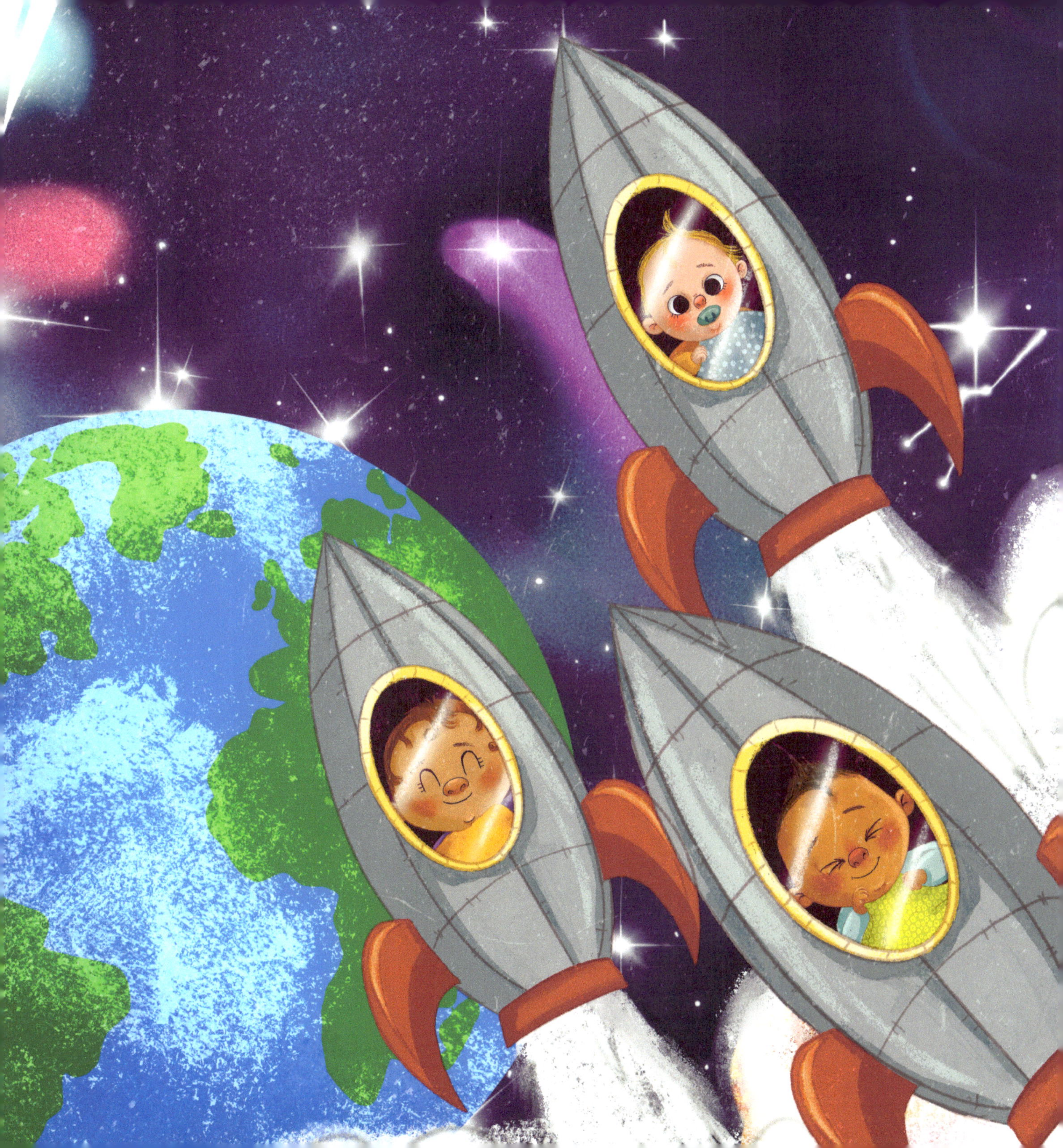

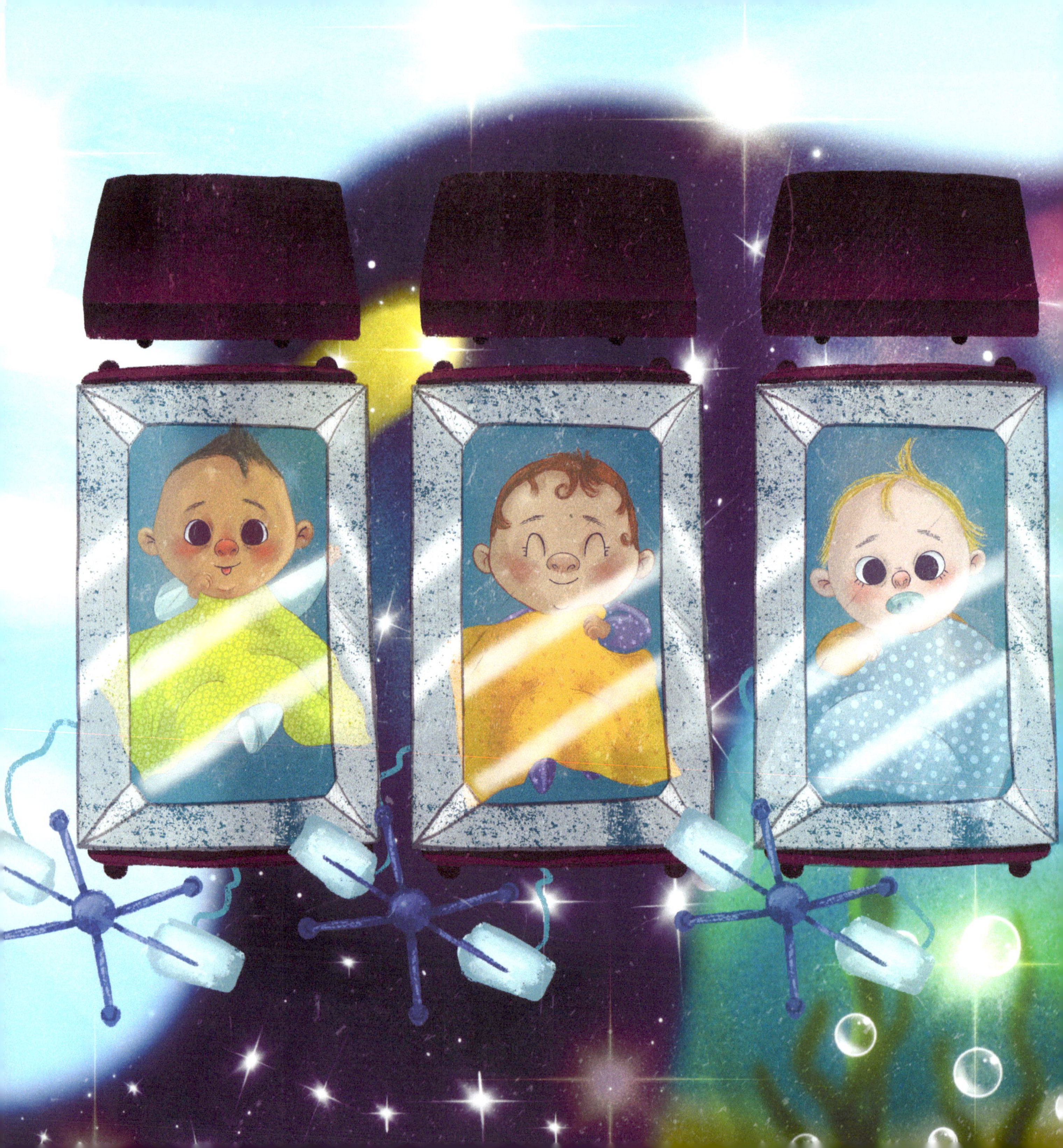

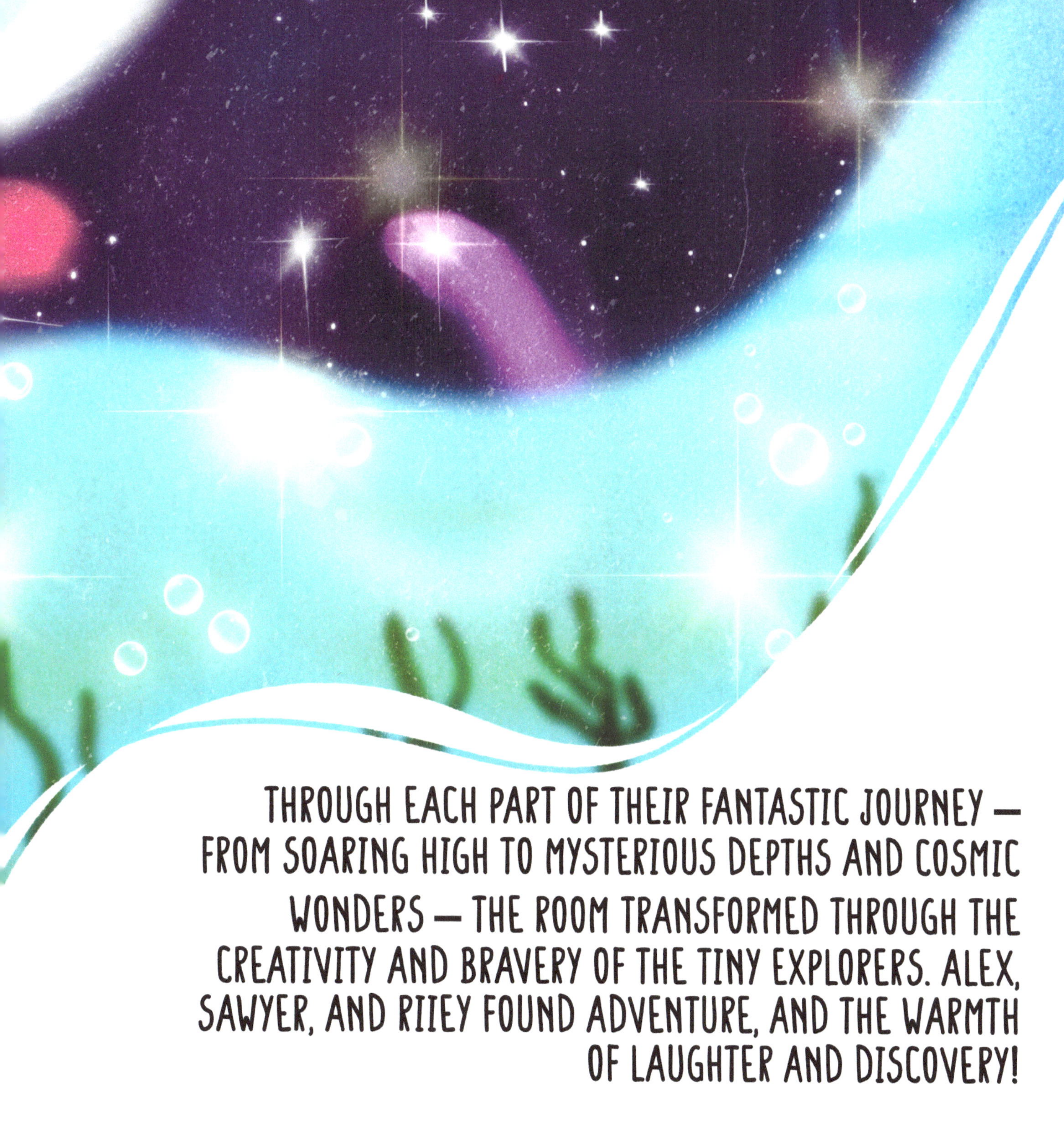

THROUGH EACH PART OF THEIR FANTASTIC JOURNEY —
FROM SOARING HIGH TO MYSTERIOUS DEPTHS AND COSMIC
WONDERS — THE ROOM TRANSFORMED THROUGH THE
CREATIVITY AND BRAVERY OF THE TINY EXPLORERS. ALEX,
SAWYER, AND RIIEY FOUND ADVENTURE, AND THE WARMTH
OF LAUGHTER AND DISCOVERY!

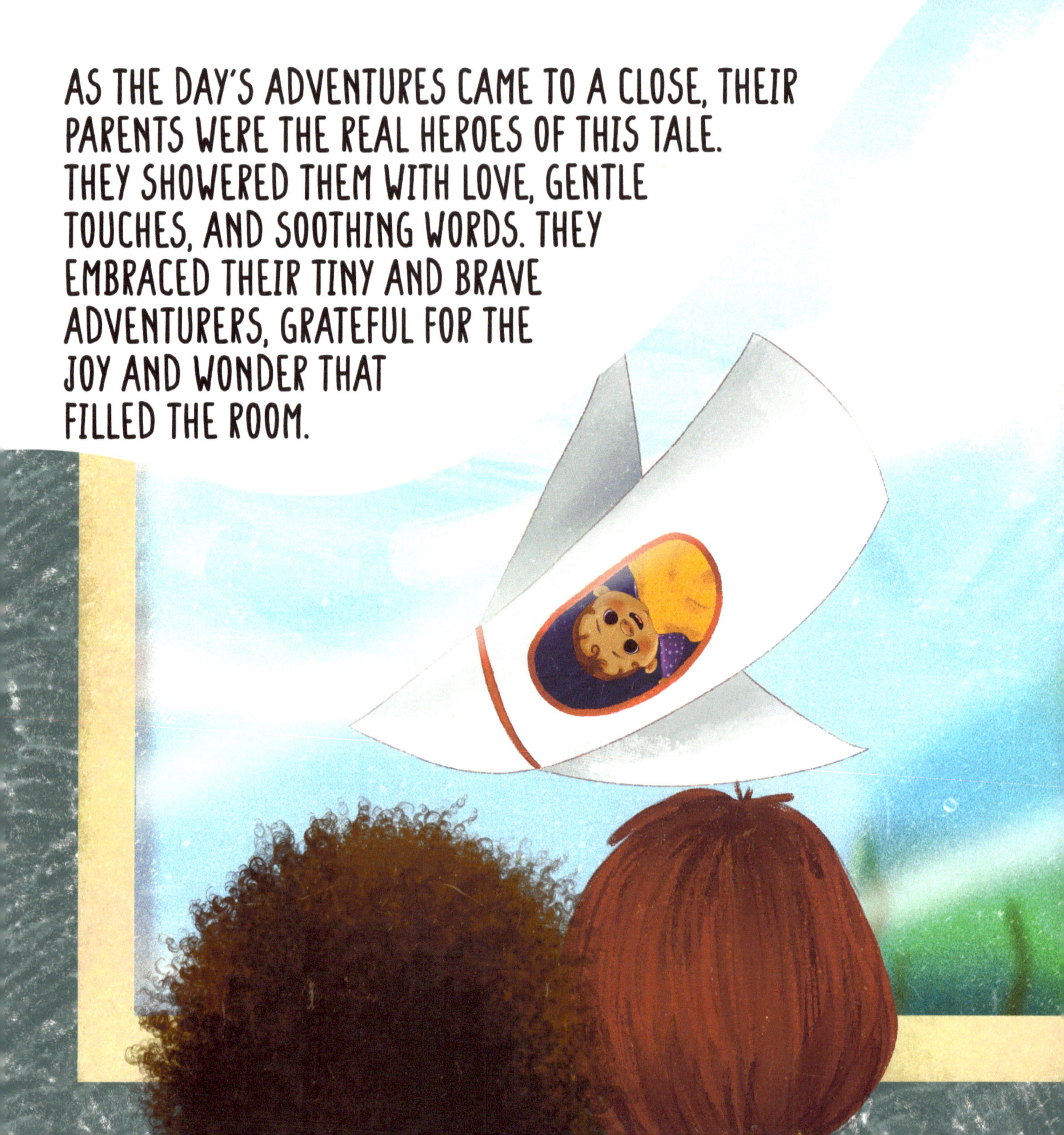

AS THE DAY'S ADVENTURES CAME TO A CLOSE, THEIR PARENTS WERE THE REAL HEROES OF THIS TALE. THEY SHOWERED THEM WITH LOVE, GENTLE TOUCHES, AND SOOTHING WORDS. THEY EMBRACED THEIR TINY AND BRAVE ADVENTURERS, GRATEFUL FOR THE JOY AND WONDER THAT FILLED THE ROOM.

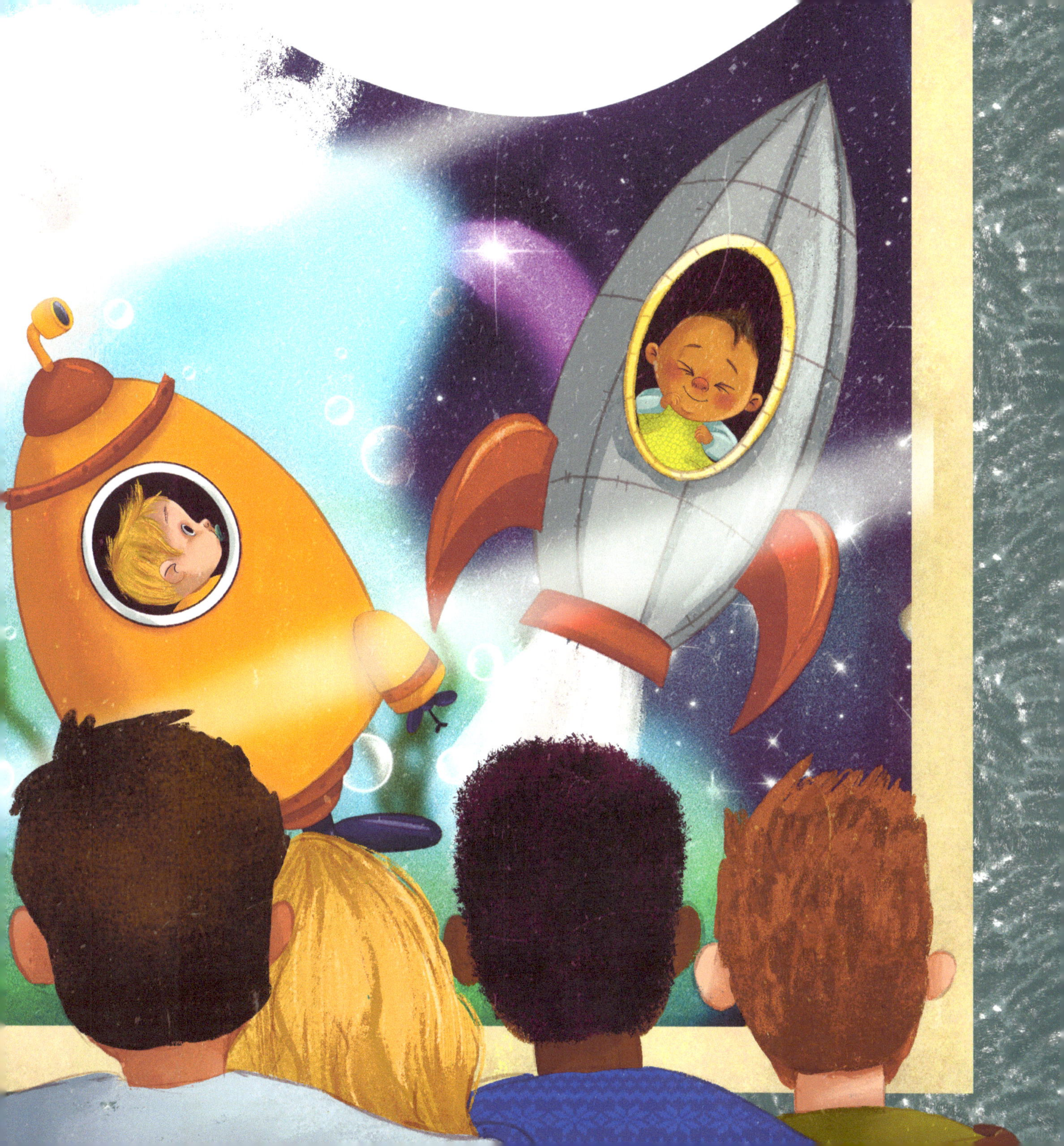

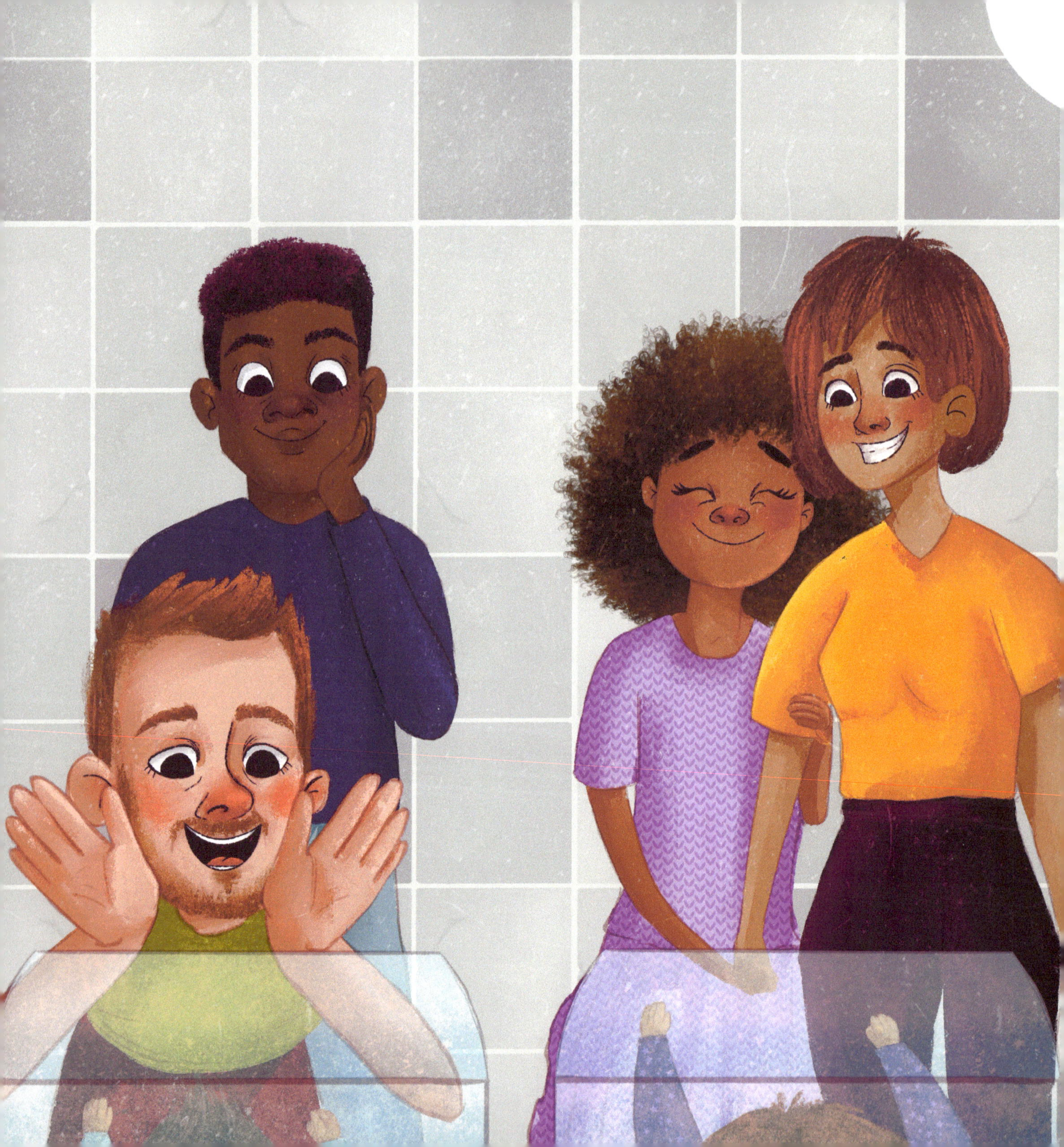

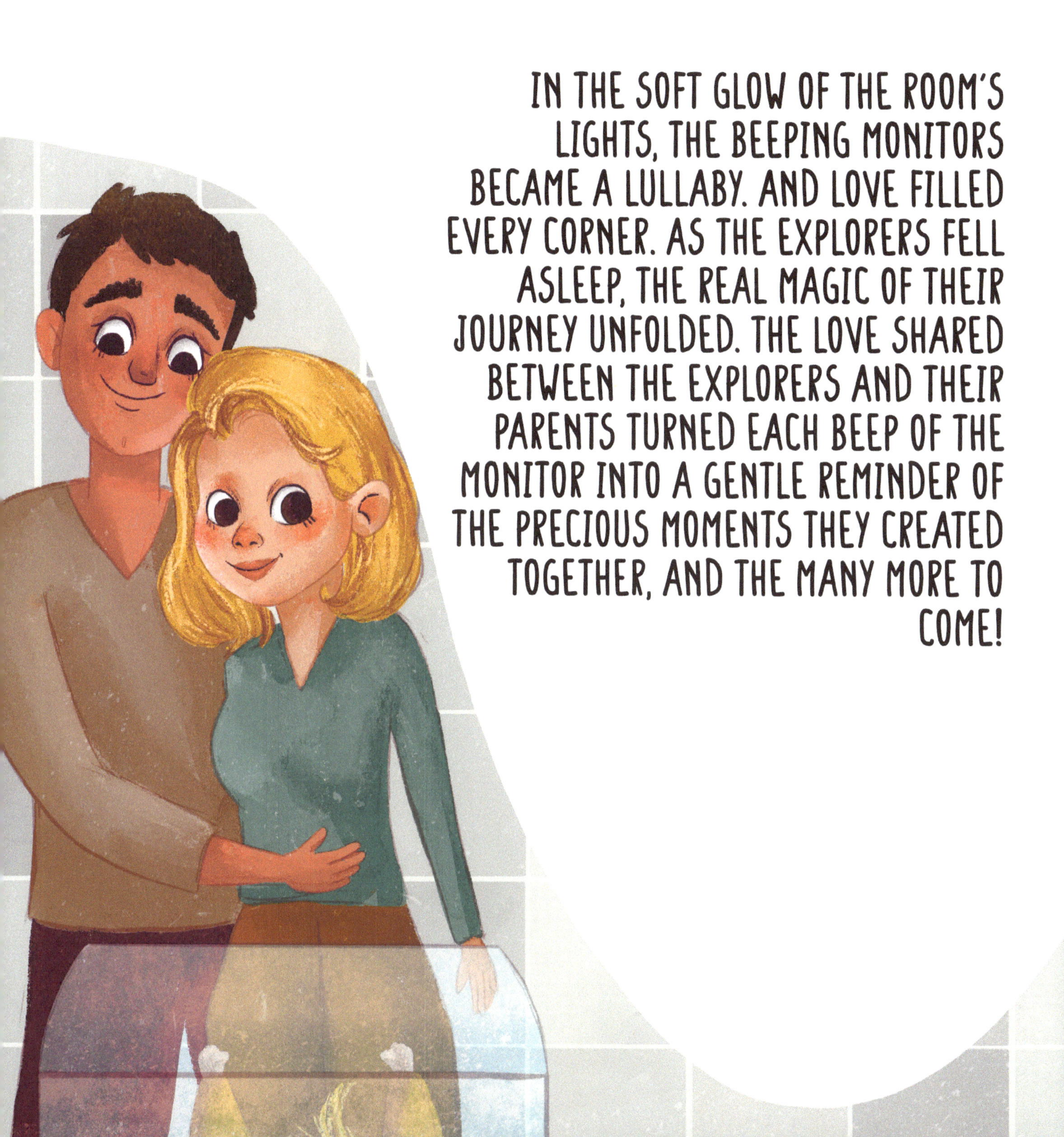

IN THE SOFT GLOW OF THE ROOM'S LIGHTS, THE BEEPING MONITORS BECAME A LULLABY. AND LOVE FILLED EVERY CORNER. AS THE EXPLORERS FELL ASLEEP, THE REAL MAGIC OF THEIR JOURNEY UNFOLDED. THE LOVE SHARED BETWEEN THE EXPLORERS AND THEIR PARENTS TURNED EACH BEEP OF THE MONITOR INTO A GENTLE REMINDER OF THE PRECIOUS MOMENTS THEY CREATED TOGETHER, AND THE MANY MORE TO COME!

Now here is a space to tell your NICU story!

Name _______________

Birthday

Weight

Length

(Place a photo of your baby here!)

Who are some of the Doctors and Nurses supporting Baby and You?

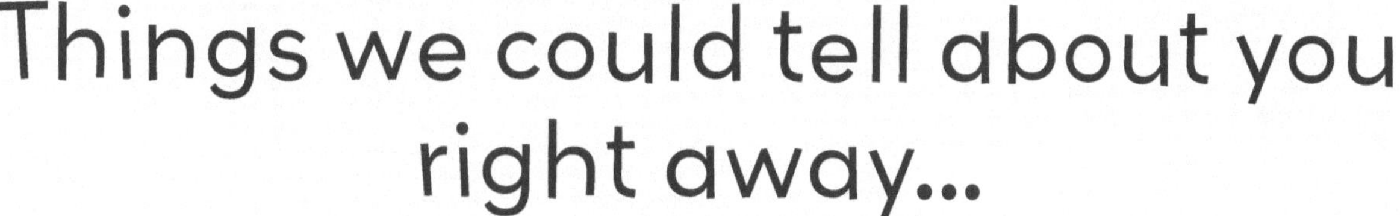

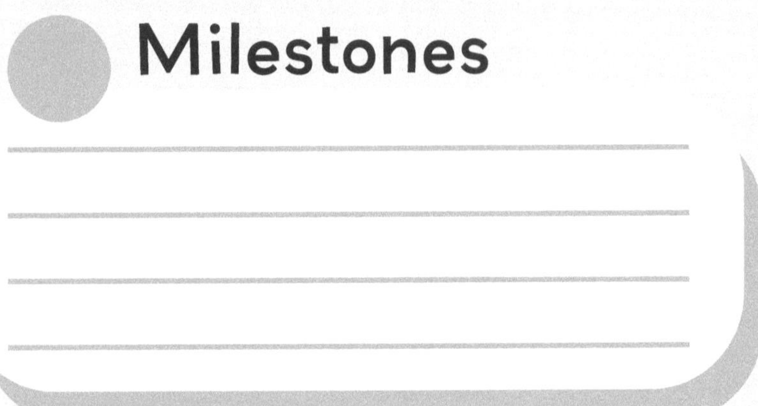

Milestones

Baby Likes

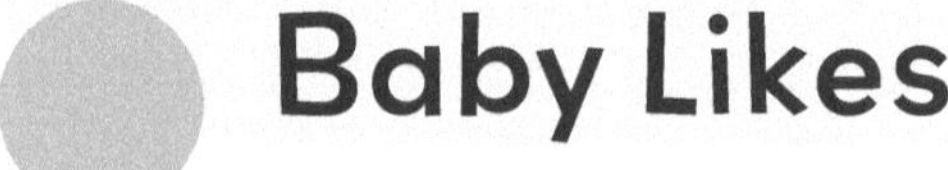

Baby Dislikes

What are some of your thoughts and feelings?

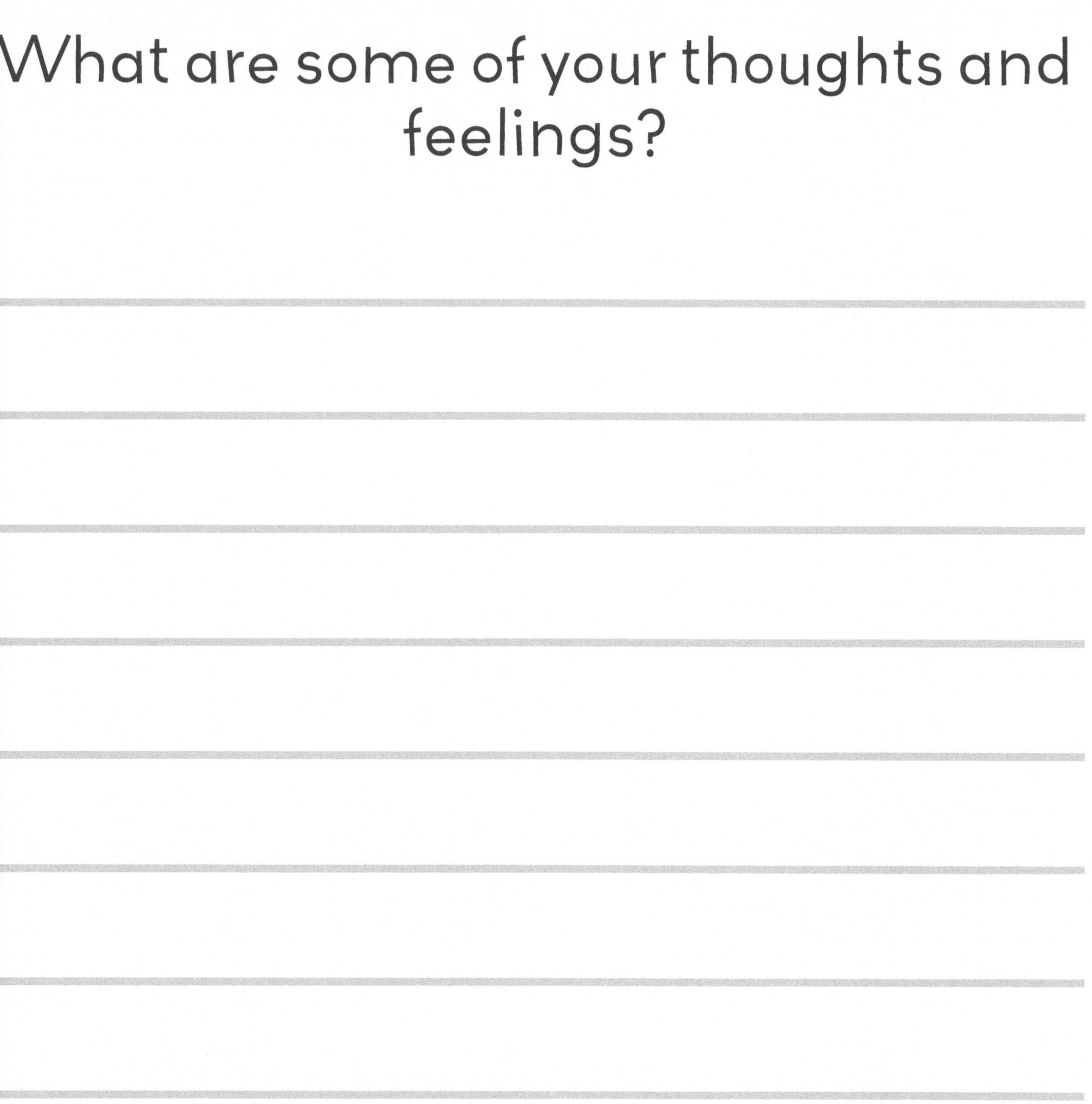

What does it feel like to hold you...

What I see when I look in your eyes...

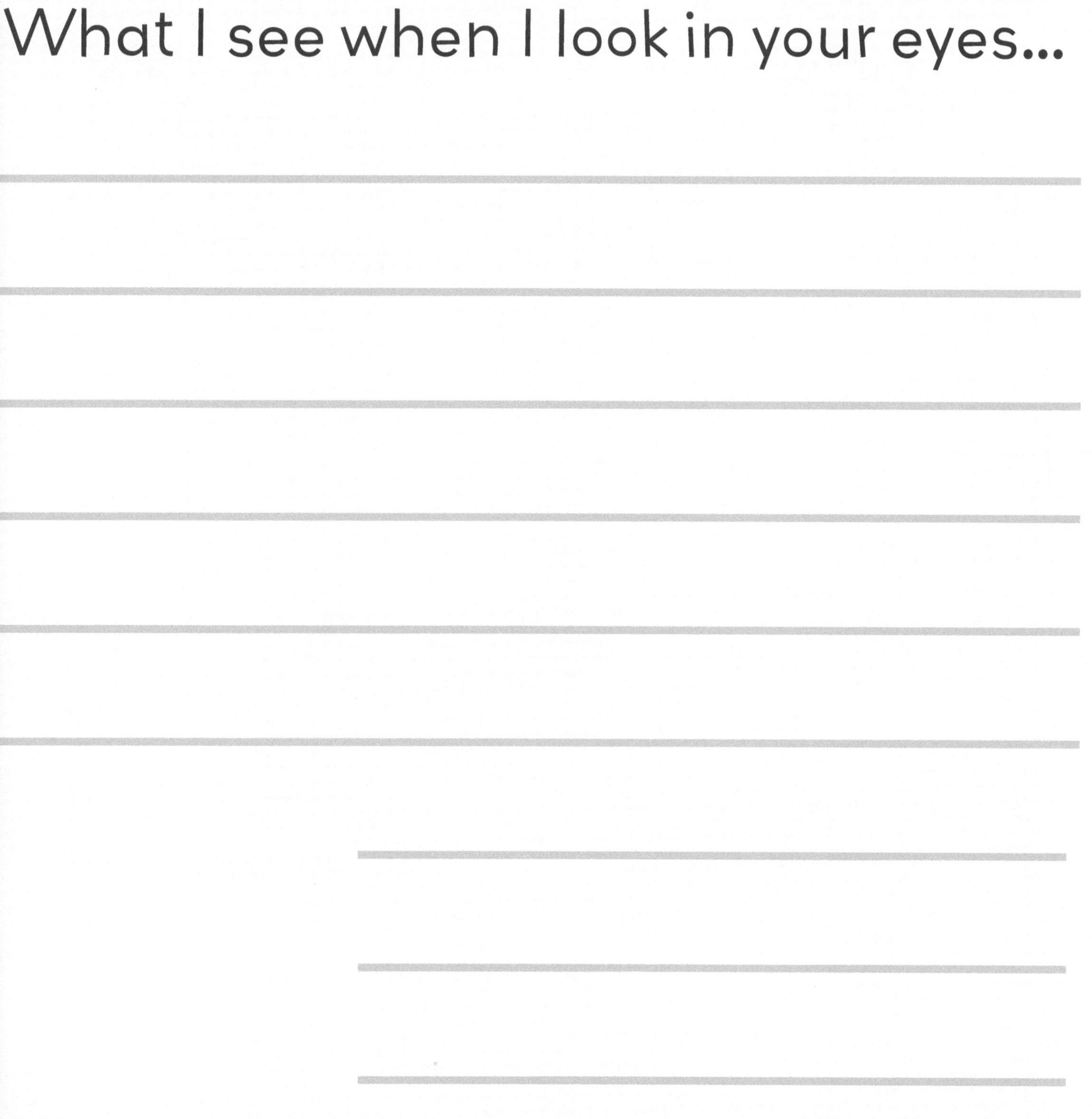

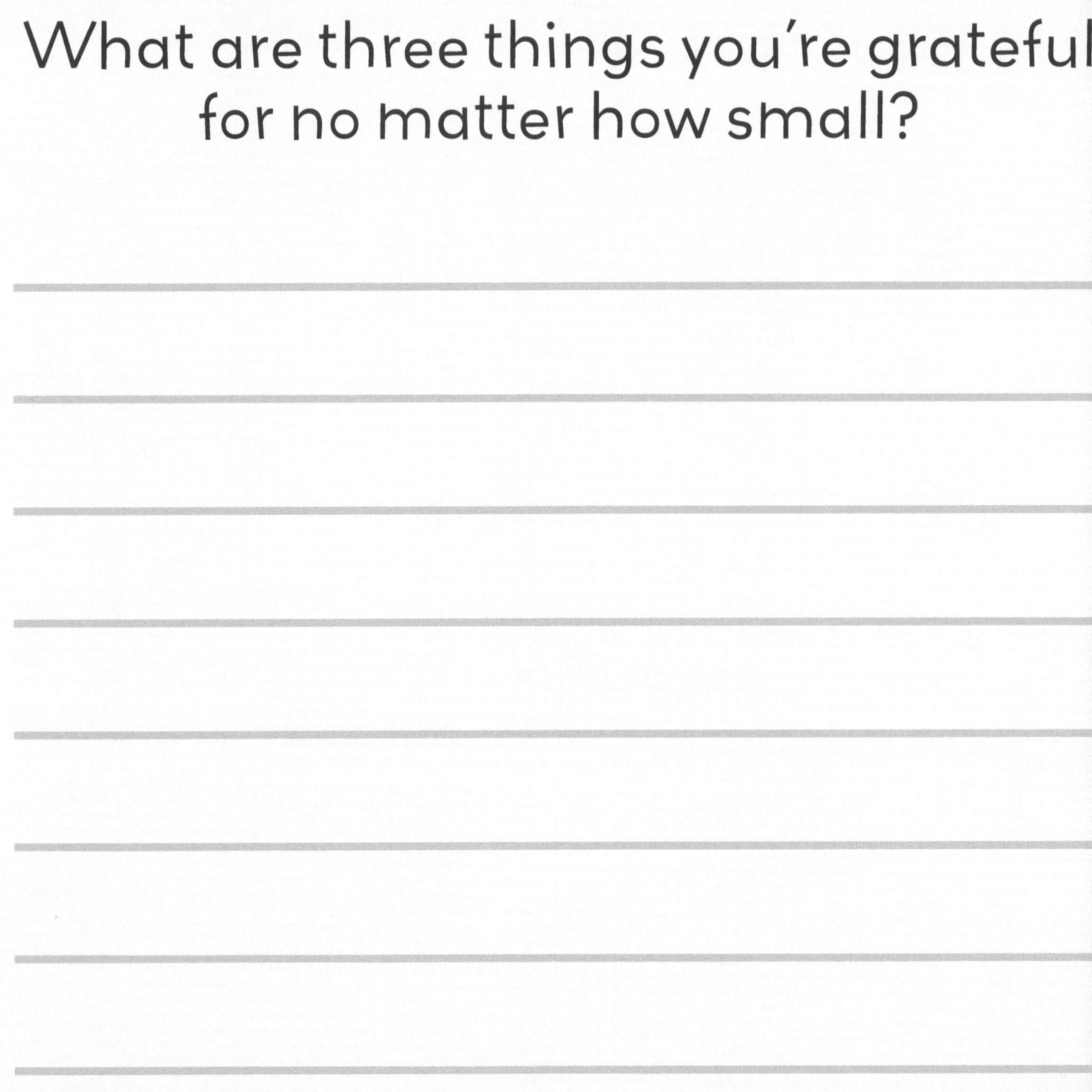

What are three things you're grateful for no matter how small?

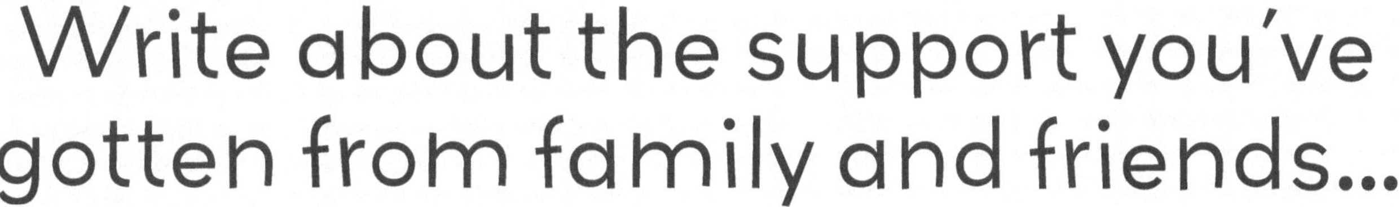

Write about the support you've gotten from family and friends...

Reflect on what you've learned about yourself, your baby, resilience during your time in the NICU...

Write a letter to your baby...

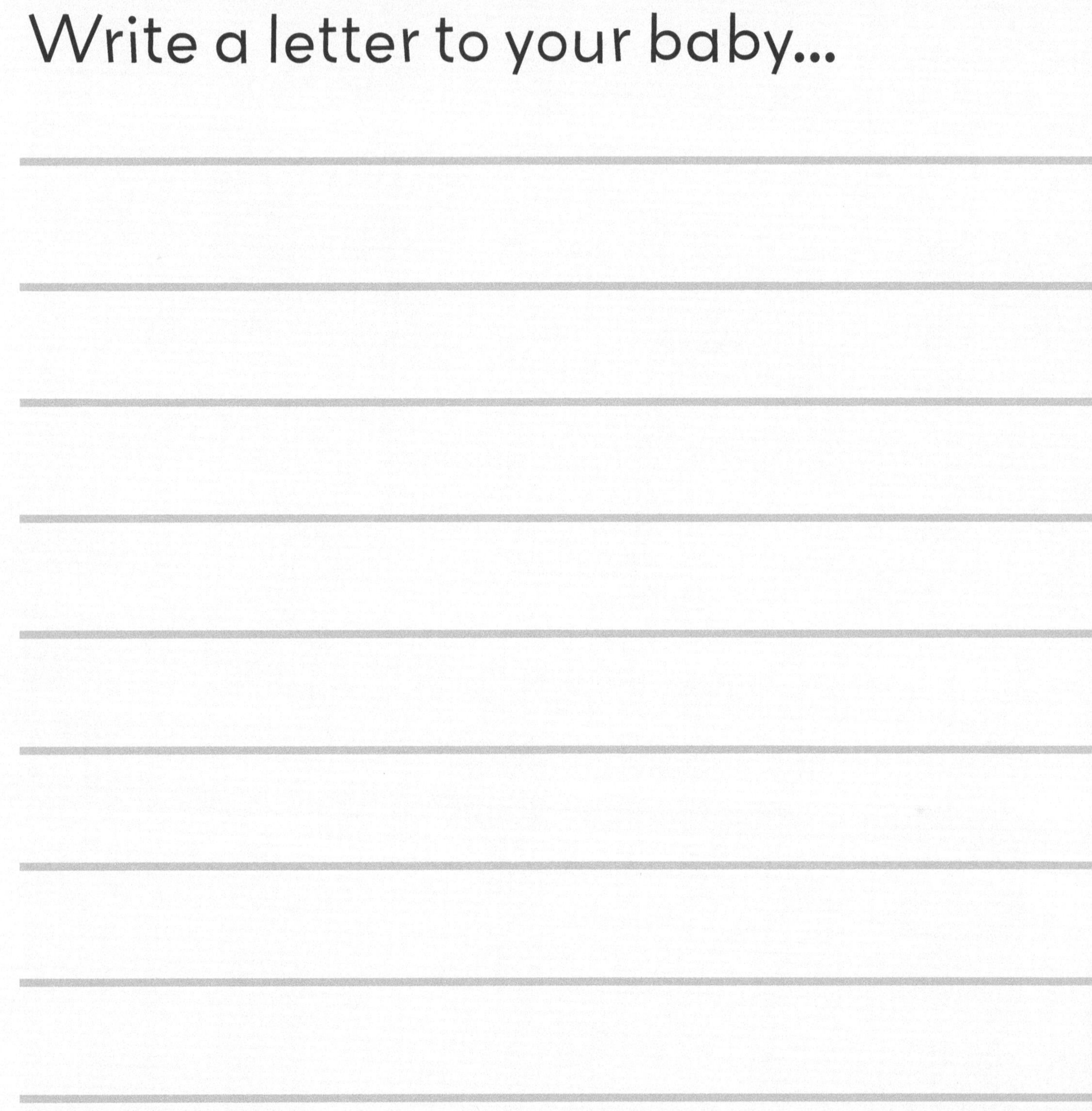

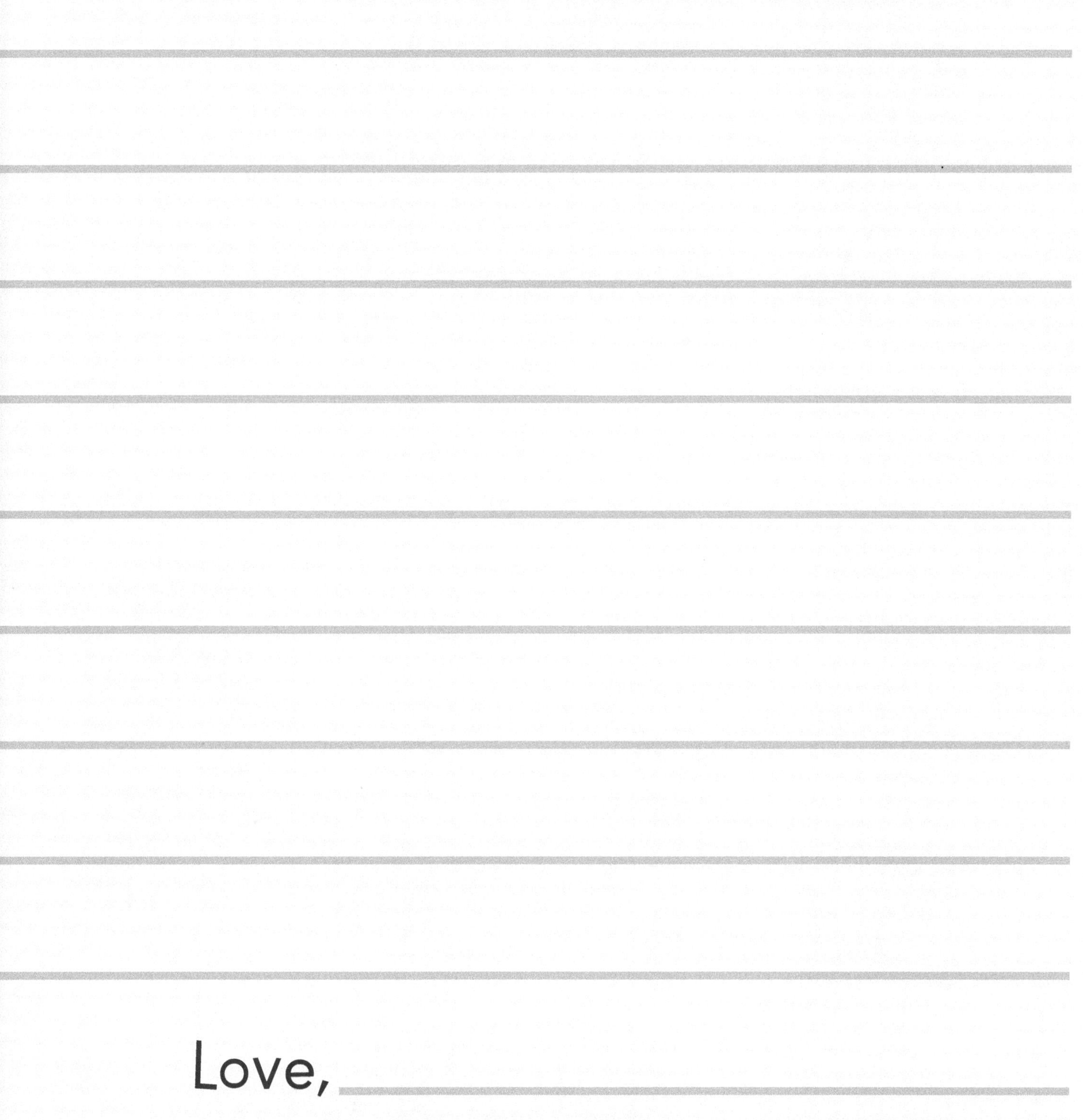
Love,

You Came Home On

How we felt...

Length of Stay

Discharge Weight

Discharge Length

(Place a photo of your baby at home!)

Home at Last!

www.ingramcontent.com/pod-product-compliance
Lightning Source LLC
Chambersburg PA
CBHW040200240726
48664CB00002B/771